See Me Now or See Me Later

A Physical Therapist's Guide to living a Stress Less Life

Dorshena M. Pittman

Printed in the United States of America

First Printing, 2018

ISBN: 13:978-0-692-18460-8

Please note: The opinions in this book are my own, and every effort has been made to include accurate information, but further research and the advice of a professional is highly recommended.

ACKNOWLEDGEMENTS

My sincerest appreciation to those who have gone before me. Those who have just by their example shown that it is possible. It's my turn up and I'm proud to have made it here!!!

Angie T. your continued inquiries about my book helped me to finish strong!

Michelle B. I did it! Your monitoring my progress let me know there was no stopping this train!

Darren V. coming up with the name of this book after I shared my vision, lit a fire that couldn't be quenched!

My book cover designer, business logo designer, and editor - you all are the best!

DEDICATION

To my heirs: my firstborn Benjamin, my only Naomi, my genius Jonathan, my baby David. I can only hope that I have made you proud and inspired you to "be one of the best!"

To my loving parents who laid the foundation and support that helped me to be who I am today, I am grateful!

To my family, friends, and strangers who have encouraged me through the years -Thank You. I did It.!!!

To those who have felt overwhelmed and stressed beyond your ability to endure it, I hope that this book inspires you and re- directs your life. You belong here, so be encouraged and be well!

Table of Contents

INTRODUCTION

"I am fearfully and wonderfully made and that I know quite well."

What fascinating and powerful words.

Can you imagine the impact they would have if we really believed them?

Imagine and consider the power of these words to change the effects of broken promises, wounding words, and situations out of our control. Such matters could cause pain, insecurity, and self-doubt.

These words (I am fearfully and wonderfully made) repeated until believed would cause the negative intent to run into a wall, a shield, that causes weapons to crumble.

Genuine peace can be found as we embrace God's thoughts concerning us as our own.

My intent is to share with you lessons from my life path until present.

Who I am now is a result of who God has been to and in me. I can remember making decisions that would have caused my life to go down a different trail, but for various reasons, I landed here.

Having practiced as a physical therapist in Louisiana and Texas for 20 + years, my perspective on life has been influenced by the patients and family members I have treated. The settings (acute, long term acute, skilled nursing facilities, inpatient rehab, and home health) have afforded me the unique opportunity to apply my skillset on the job and off. The abilities that come naturally to us, but that have to be relearned after injury, are the needs that I have continually been assigned to help restore. Imagine having to re-learn how to roll over, sit, stand, and walk again. I have been brought to tears watching a leg move again that initially after injury, had absolutely no movement. As rewarding as it has been, I would rather an individual See Me Now for education on preventing having a stroke, rather than to See Me Later for stroke rehabilitation.

As a physical therapist, I have been allowed to meet individuals of various nationalities, ages, and backgrounds. People have had a varied list of diagnoses both common and different, though one thing is true. Healing all had the same basic truth. The internal systems that worked together were what had to be restored. Those organs, nerves, muscles, and systems all connected the same. Blood vessels provided oxygen, nerves stimulated muscles, and the spinal cord relayed information to the brain.

Automatic processes continued without permission, and so much else that allows us to be our uniquely and wonderfully made selves. The realization that the restoration of all patients involved the same knowledge and physical contact allows me to share my insight with you confidently.

CHAPTER ONE
Follow The Footprints

Thinking of my parents makes me smile. They set an example of a loving, devoted, and God-fearing couple. They loved not only their children but people they knew and didn't know. They tried to set an example of living that was respectable not only to the community but each other.

Memories of dad telling a joke which made the cashier laugh were awe-inspiring to me; that he had the power to cause someone else's demeanor to be lifted. Strangers were not immune to dad's ease of conversation and humor. I can remember being prideful of his ability to draw others into his world of kindness and compassion for others. He had the ability to play the piano by ear and harmonize when singing. I truly believe my love of harmony is from hearing him blend in so well to the background or in leading songs. In my eyes, he could do no wrong (except when he punished me that one time for calling a boy on the phone before I was allowed to do so).

Mom loved dad and her kids so much. She was his constant companion such that it was shocking to see him in the community without her. She took pleasure in having her kids clean, dressed, and waiting at the door when dad arrived home from work. We would fight over who got to kiss him first. Mom kept her home clean and presentable which set the example that I enforce in my home.

Mom faithfully attended a weekly prayer meeting (Bible band). It was a group of ladies who met at different churches to pray together. Mom always took her kids with her. At one of those meetings, I recall an older lady saying to me, "God's going to use you one day." As a child, I didn't really understand what that meant but those words resonated with me and I never forgot them. At times in my life, they come back to my remembrance vividly. They were a piece of a puzzle that helped bring me to where I am today. When confronted with situations in life, I would always remember that God was going to use me one day.

I knew there was a plan for my life early on because we were taught to respect our elders. This elder who was part of this committed, passionate group of ladies who sought and looked up to God had spoken this word into my life. I am forever grateful for her decision to share those words with me. Mom's decision to expose me to an atmosphere of Godly reverence brought me into contact with someone whose words have encouraged me and pieced together the plan for my life. There are those in my life who influenced me even though they didn't know it. Some had a greater impact than others. The evidence of that is the changes in my life that were inspired by their life. Others I have simply admired, respected, or took note of qualities that were unique to that individual. The ones whose influences stand out are still with me and are practiced by me today.

One such one was an aunt of mine. As a young teen, I remember her teaching me to hold my abdominal muscles in tightly. I practiced this technique through adulthood. Many times others would take note of my physique not knowing that I was simply practicing my aunt's advice. She taught me the control that's possible with practice. I practiced this technique and taught others who were interested. Knowing the ability I had to maintain the appearance I desired was not lost on physique only.

It was consistently choosing to follow her advice that produced the results I desired. Only knowing the information would not have yielded results. No. Putting the knowledge into practice regularly produced results. There must be action connected with the desire for a certain outcome to manifest. I see results when I consistently make choices to eat healthily and exercise. When I choose not to eat right and exercise, I don't see the muscle tone I long for. Desiring results without the actions to achieve them are void. Let's get results!

Charlotte (name changed) was another person who made an impression on me that lasts until this day. I never saw her looking unkempt. You know, dressing mismatched or in "these are my cleaning up clothes." Whether I dropped by to visit at her home or saw her out and about in the community, she always presented as though "she woke up like this." "Like this" was always presentable and stylish. I only knew one other person who always was dressed to impress. Both people were ladies who had nothing to prove to me. They simply appeared never to be caught off guard, or needed to tidy up before opening their door to greet you. I liked their presentation and used their images as motivation to at least present well in the community.

I remember having a dream as a young girl of myself climbing up a ladder. The ladder was based on the earth, but it went up into the cloud. Symbolically I knew I was going to be with God. Before I could reach the top where the ladder and clouds met, I remember being told that God needed me on the earth. I couldn't go at that time. I couldn't continue the journey to enter in or go pass the clouds because God needed me on the earth and was going to use me. It was another marker, another directive that helped point me to the knowledge that there was something I needed to do here on earth.

Growing up, I walked through life carefree. I can only attribute this to my Godly parents who intentionally or not allowed me to just be. Being me came without prep or planning. It just seemed that life happened to me. I, in return, flowed with it and said yes when opportunities arose. Whether excelling in academic or extracurricular activities, it just seemed that I went with the current. Considering that now I am considered a peacemaker, the foundation obviously was well laid.

I remember in middle school having the only physical fight in my life; it was with a classmate. I recall being on top with my fist lifted to exact a hurling punch. It was as though the Lord himself or an angel held my fist in place. I honestly was positioned with my fist held high and unable to bring it down to make contact. The teacher separated us, and I got in trouble (even though I didn't take her out). I always wonder if it was because the peacemaker framework was already unfolding.

The unwillingness to cause harm but having the ability to do so was and has been evident in many situations. Just because the power is within our control for vengeance or punishment does not lend itself to outcomes that will not bring regret. I offer the mindset that having the power to do so, and not welding it is much more authoritative and empowering. It also brings peace that the urge was overridden by the choice to do no harm.

Simply put, choosing peace is rewarding to the recipient and the giver.

I am one of five siblings. I always loved holidays growing up. Holidays involved going from one relative's home to the next. There was always a house full of people, and I grew to love and prefer this atmosphere. We would get to meet up with aunts, uncles, cousins, neighbors... everyone was welcome. As kids, we played with abandon.

We also used to meet every Sunday after church at my grandparent's home. Once again it was an opportunity to hang out with family. Grandma made the best homemade ice cream. Unfortunately, she took the recipe to her grave.

My parents were also a member of a social and pleasure club. This group would meet monthly, and the meeting places would rotate. I only have fond memories of those meetings.

One of my cousins chose to become a doctor. Her decision influenced mine to consider a future in the medical field. My first choice in college was computer science. I made A's in the field, and my professor tried to encourage me to pursue it. I enjoyed science and preferred to work with people, so working with computers just didn't hold my interest. Next, medical technology was an option. When I found out I'd be handling others' urine, I decided I just couldn't do it. Physical Therapy practically fell into my lap as I found the field while browsing through a roommate's college catalog. My pursuit in the field was hindered when I applied the first time to P.T. school and was denied. I needed to have volunteer or work hours in the field. This was to make sure this was truly the field that you wanted to practice in. The competition was fierce to get into school, so the school tried to filter out those who were going to finish the program from those who were applying and were not certain that this was the profession for them. You could only apply to P.T. school annually. I decided to try the military after getting rejected. Every medical field I applied to was closed. There was no place for me. I believe this was God intervening so that I would stay on course to becoming a Physical Therapist. After volunteering, I reapplied and was accepted to P.T. school. It has been a perfect fit for me.

As an adult, my focus has been to exist with a heart that is free of bitterness. I have seen through the eyes of my occupation, individuals deal with the stress that accompanied their choices. My goal is to examine my heart, motives, intent, and ensure that my choices are from a pure place. I self-reflect as to whether I am holding anyone hostage with unforgiveness, envy or jealousy. If any of these are evident, I choose to let it go. I make conscious decisions to serve or be willing to serve others so as to remain humble. I believe that it is easier to get up from a lower place than to fall from an exalted mindset.

I thought I had sufficiently checked my heart. One day I heard my pastor preach on unforgiveness; immediately, I began to consider if there was anyone I hadn't forgiven. The only situation I could think of involved a former co-worker. Our relationship hadn't ended well. It had been years since we had worked together. We seldom (maybe once or twice) had come into contact with each other. When we did, we maintained our distance. I made a decision that I would sincerely hug her if I ever saw her again. My goal was not to let anyone or thing clog my heart so that the flow between God and I would not be blocked. Instead, the blessings would flow unhindered.

Approximately two months later on a cruise ship, she and I met up. When we recognized each other, we hugged as though we were family. We talked and caught up on each other's lives as though nothing ever happened. We have not had contact since then, nor do we need to. My heart was free. Having clean hands, and a clean heart and a passion to completely fill the assignment on my life allows the vision to be written and make it plain to see.

At this point, I feel compelled to complete this task (book writing) and to initiate the next (motivational speaking). There have been recent tugs and pushes that have convinced me this is indeed the correct path for me.

In July, while doing what I enjoy doing – shopping; someone I didn't know began speaking to me. I was unprepared because she approached me from behind, then came to my right, then in front. She initially complemented me on the outfit I had tried on and mentioned the word "royalty." She continued to speak and communicate inspiring words to me. The words that I recall most were "there are words in you that people need to hear." She spoke these words a few times. She also said there are books you need to write and not just one book. This was especially significant to me. I would tell my friends about my plan to talk to people about a certain subject. I felt I had A, B, and C to say, then I would be done. Her words had a great impact on me. I sensed a compelling that I needed to move forward with the next chapter of my life. Of course, there are always obstacles that will arise to hinder the process. We must resist these forces and keep the vision as a priority. Without it, our plans will perish (fade away).

Thank God for the Holy Spirit who will bring things back to our remembrance.

CHAPTER TWO
Uniquely You

You and others like you have things in common. That commonality does not take away from the fact that you are unique. No other mammal is a match for you. Your fingerprints are yours and yours alone. There have been times that someone will say, "You look just like so and so." I always ask to see a picture of that person, but a picture has never been available. The times that a person said this in person was simply because we had similar eye color and complexion. Never a true match! I must admit I wasn't surprised. I fully embrace the fact that I am uniquely made. It affirms my particular purpose on earth. I encourage you to hold fast and true that you are wonderfully made.

I challenge you to consider body mechanics. Have you ever tried to rise to stand while leaning backward? No one as of yet has been able to do so. I believe it supports the mindset that in order to move forward, you must move forward. Looking or leaning backward hinders forward progress. What's behind you should propel you to improve, to build on, to do better. The future is waiting for you to rise to the occasion.

In a standing position, try leaning your body weight on one leg then picking that leg up to step forward. Continue maintaining your body weight on the same leg and attempt to move forward. Not possible! You must unweight yourself to move forward. Now lean off of that leg to the other side and step forward, easy right? You deliberately took the weight off of your extremity thereby allowing yourself the freedom to pick up the unweighted leg and step forward.

So often we get stuck and weighted down that we forget to unweight ourselves. You have to realize that this is too heavy a matter, and it's weighing you down. Look at the matter from a different perspective. What can I do to shift this so that I can be free to move forward? Is it that important, but difficult to manage alone? If so, can someone else help carry the load? Often times when I am working with patients, they may push with one side of their body and hinder me from helping them to sit straight up. I have to give them directions, encourage, and assist them to let me move their body for them. It is not always easy but rewarding when we work together.

There are times when a patient has a fear of falling. It is difficult to get them to lean forward. Because of previous falls, there is a powerful reluctance to lean forward. This fear can be debilitating and may keep a person from doing what previously came easily. I now understand and can relate to this feeling. While on vacation celebrating my birthday, I went into the Airbnb we were renting to retrieve a jacket for my mom and slipped down a flight of stairs. There was no rail, so there was nothing to stop my fall. It was the most frightening experience I have ever had. I pushed past the pain and bruising the next day and went zip lining. After all, it was my birthday celebration! I found myself asking family to walk with me down the steps after that experience. Even when I returned home, I would hold on to the wall or rails while climbing the stairs. At some point, I decided to walk down steps without holding on. That experience helped me to relate to my patients' concerns and to let them know I could relate. It gave us a common experience to bond over. There are others who can help each of us shift the burdens and weights that we carry to lessen the stress we feel. We must, however, choose to move forward.

Where does fear come from? Does it come from a place of knowing, the memory of what happened last time, or from lack of knowledge? For example: how many people associate a skeleton with a fearful response? The truth is, it is an astounding exhibition of how intricately we have been designed. Without the boney framework, we would not be whole. Whether big or small, young or old, short or tall, from the Western or Eastern hemisphere, all humans have the same basic boney structure. It is to that structure that muscles attach and allow us the freedom and ability to move. Parents have instructed kids to drink milk so as to have strong bones. Calcium is stored in bones and is important for nerves and muscles to work properly. When viewing a skeleton, some shrink away in fear. Realize it is the foundation of the uniquely made you. It makes it possible for us to move, and it protects and shapes the human body.

With knowledge, we can move from a state of fear to a place of empowerment.

Did you know that nose hairs are the most sensitive hairs on our body? Why do you think this is so? I believe it is because there has to be a filter to decrease the risk of particles entering our respiratory system and affecting our ability to breathe. Awesome, isn't it?

Have you thought about the fact that the skull shapes the head and face? So, if you don't like the shape of your head, realize it's the skull's fault.:) It also serves to protect the brain and keeps the brain stationary. The brain controls the rate of our breathing, it is the biggest user of oxygen and suffers if the oxygen supply is decreased. It's important to keep it protected, right? The ribs protect the vital organs (heart and lungs) and aid in breathing. The spine allows you to stand upright and to balance. The bones contain bone marrow that produces blood cells which provide oxygen that in turn provides the energy we need. Do you know that the human body is made up of 206 bones? The infant body contains even more, though some fuse as the body grows. Did you know that the lungs are the only organ that are exposed to the external environment? Lungs are vulnerable to bronchitis and emphysema. We must, therefore, make decisions to keep them healthy.

Why do you think some lives are so uniquely different from others? Some would say it's because of nature. What comes naturally to us, or what we naturally choose to do? One person's decision may produce life. By that I mean a positive outcome, success, or rewards. That choice very well may be influenced by the way a person was raised. What comes natural to one person may be to be kind. In return kindness comes back to them. Another may decide to be tolerant and forgiving and the same comes back to them. Someone else may choose (possibly due to examples observed while growing up) to be generous. Maybe in return acts of generosity may be the normal product that returns to that individual.

A person who models him or herself after the principle of seed sowing (giving) would likely be a recipient of their deeds. Whether that person passed the harvest on to others or not, I believe there will be a return on the investment. Each of us who gives should do so with the knowledge and expectation that there will be growth from that which was given. Their life decisions will undoubtedly affect others' perception of the benefit of giving, and bring to the giver the ultimate satisfaction of investing with or without expectation of harvest. Be encouraged to give just because endorphins released from doing so just simply feel good.

What if one was raised in an environment such that what seems to come naturally is lost and lacks positive reinforcement? The natural responses for this person may be to shelter their goods or to hide their treasures. Could it be that a person who always has their hand out to receive does so because everything was always taken from them?

A reaction from living in lack could also be a tendency to take. This person may never know the joy of giving because their natural responses are to be a recipient. There is a precedent for kids to be self-centered and to not know the joy of being a giver because being a receiver is their norm.

It is a choice to be generous. Generosity can be through words to inspire others. It can be through a smile in passing or a touch to acknowledge another's existence. The giving is most freeing though when no expectations are attached to the giving. In that way, there is no disappointment when the giving may not be acknowledged. More times than not others respond to gestures given freely. Take a moment to give a nod, a smile, or a greeting first, and feel your self unweighting.

Consider the person who seems to be neither moving forward or backward; same routine day in and day out; same breakfast, same basic ingredients for lunch and dinner. Meals are approximately the same time every day. Movements follow the same pattern.

Someone once told me that they never leave the house. No open window blinds. No sunshine. The sad part is that the person became content with the same daily routine. In response, her muscles were weakened, her endurance was limited, and her desire for more was stunted. This state became natural - her norm. It limited her interactions with others and her awareness of what was available to improve her status. Access to means to help her life become more productive was stunted. She expressed no joy.

Though different regions have different lengths of seasons, seasons are generally accepted to be normal. There are changes that happen naturally through seasons. If the seasonal change is resisted or is not acknowledged, one can become vulnerable. Environmental changes, if welcomed can bring benefits which otherwise are lost to the observer. Summer usually requires different attire than winter. Fall exhibits patterns that are beautiful to experience.

Choosing to remain in one season or another while changes happen around you limits a person from enjoying the beauty that life offers.

Stagnant living, or being involved in seasonal changes which do you choose?

Being intact involves the mind, body, and Spirit being connected and operating efficiently. As we reach a certain stage in life, our awareness of the need to be at peace is sharpened. Some focus more on being fit physically. There are those who spend hours in the gym only to neglect relationships in their lives that should be prioritized. Others are intellectuals who research and study and lose out on social interactions with others who may benefit from the knowledge the intellect has attained. Still, others spend time focused wholly on the spiritual and forget to share love with those who are not like minded. When systems are intact, it is easy to JUST BE and reflect the light of being at peace. Neglecting the whole can cause a person to miss the joy of living a balanced life.

A stress-less life involves identifying and fulfilling opportunities for wholeness. Choosing to prioritize (what's most important), to be good with you, and sharing with others leads to a win-win outcome. No man is an island, so be quick to listen, slow to speak, and empowered in knowing you belong here!

It would seem that as a person matures, life becomes easier. A child often falls as he or she is learning to walk. The ability to stand and step forward for some comes sooner and easier than others. Some may learn quicker because they're tired of falling and the pain that accompanies the fall.

Even so, as an adult, some find their footing, their passion, their purpose sooner rather than later. The pain of falling or failing may be an incentive to try harder, choose a different means or foundation to help achieve a standing position. Prior to standing, trunk or core control is essential. Self-worth, an "I belong here, I make a difference" mindset is necessary. One must know this in order to build a foundation to move forward.

When attending an event, I assume that empty seats are potentially mine. If it is not obviously another person's seat, I assume it can be mine. My approach exemplifies that mindset. I say that to say existing in life is enhanced by the belief that you were born for a purpose. You were allowed to see life and exist at this time because there is a reason for you to be here. So walk like it. Respect others, and expect to be respected. Be wise and discerning, and yet confident. Know the angels are here for you as you acknowledge the creator and his plan for your life. As you embrace life, it will respond in kind. Keep your head up, keep getting up, and seize the day!

CHAPTER THREE
When Normal Goes Wrong

The American Heart Association reports that there are 800,000 Americans who suffer strokes per year, 80% of which are preventable through lifestyle changes.

Cerebrovascular disorders (CVA)/strokes represent the 3rd leading cause of death and the 2nd major cause of long-term disability. A stroke happens when blood flow and oxygen are suddenly interrupted to an area of brain tissue which then dies.

The brain is made up of left and right hemispheres. Strokes that affect the right hemisphere results in left-sided weakness and opposite-sided neglect. Strokes that affect the left hemisphere present right-sided weakness and aphasia. The artery affected will determine the clinical manifestation. The middle cerebral artery covers two-thirds of the medial surface of the cerebral hemisphere. This artery is most commonly affected by a stroke. When damage occurs in the brain, the entire brain suffers from the loss of input.

The brain is divided into lobes. The frontal lobe is the control panel. It controls cognitive function and voluntary movements, emotional expression, problem solving, memory, language, judgment, and sexual behavior. The temporal lobe is involved in primary auditory perception, vision, memory, sensory input, language, emotion, and comprehension. It is key in our being able to hear and comprehend. The parietal lobe processes taste, temperature, and touch. It is vital to process sensory information concerning the location of body parts and interpreting visual information, language, and math processing. The occipital lobe processes visual information. It allows us to understand what we see correctly.

This brief synopsis allows us a glimpse into how intricately we were made. Injury to the most minor member of our body such as the little toe is perceived by the most complex structure - the brain.

Common risk factors for stroke include high blood pressure, diabetes, high cholesterol, smoking, obesity, and lack of exercise. Blood vessels narrow and damage arteries that supply the brain. High blood pressure is the leading cause of stroke and the MOST controllable risk factor. 80% of recurring strokes are preventable with treatment and lifestyle changes.

High blood pressure or HTN is known as the "silent killer." It quietly damages blood vessels. It happens when the force of blood through your blood vessels is too high. Age, heredity, gender, race, and kidney disease are risk factors out of one's control. Modifiable risk factors - those you can change include lack of physical activity, unhealthy diet especially high in sodium, being overweight or obese, too much alcohol, sleep apnea, high cholesterol, diabetes, smoking/tobacco use, and stress.

An increase in obesity and chronic conditions such as Type 2 diabetes, high cholesterol and high blood pressure among young people could lead to greater stroke risk as they age. It could be the tip of the iceberg because complications of heart disease and chronic conditions have not caught up to them yet. Increased access to health care is important to identify the risk factor early.

Atrial fibrillation is a process that can increase stroke risk 5x; it doubles the heart-related death chance. Atrial fibrillation is a heart rhythm that allows extra blood to pool in the heart. It is caused by an abnormal heartbeat - arrhythmia. Normal heart rate is 60-100 beats/minute. In atrial fibrillation, the heart rate is fast (140-180beats/minute and irregular). The heart doesn't empty each cycle. Irregular impulses and weak contractions occur in the upper chamber of the heart (atria). The heart doesn't empty each cycle, and left over blood forms a clot which can move through the bloodstream to the brain and can cause a stroke.

Knowledge is power. So let's consider this information and be empowered. We are defenseless when we just don't know, but we're equipped to make changes once we are informed.

In all my years of treating patients and helping to restore individuals' function, there is one thing that has never happened. I have never had a grateful person say the recovery was so worth it that he or she would like to experience a stroke again. Let's make choices to reduce the risk of ever having a first stroke.

"The best stroke is the stroke you never had."
Neurologist Julius S. Latorre M.D.

Stress is the state of mental or emotional strain from adverse or very demanding circumstances (it's different for each person). Stress is felt when one has to handle more than he or she is used to. The body responds as though there is danger. Hormones are released which cause increased heart rate, faster breathing, and increased burst of energy. There is increased blood pressure, increased pulse, digestive systems slow, immune activity increases, and muscle tension increases. The increased state of alertness prevents sleep. The body is flooded with chemicals that prepare for the stress response. Consider if this system is activated daily. This is the fight or flight response. Short-term stress can be helpful but long term it is linked to various health conditions. When one is stressed out frequently, the body remains in a heightened state of stress.

Increase in the stress hormone leads to increased storage of visceral fat. Visceral fat secrets retinal binding protein which increases insulin resistance. Visceral fat can raise blood pressure quickly. Belly fat is a sign of visceral fat; fat that gathers around organs in the abdomen. This fat promotes insulin resistance and unhealthy cholesterol numbers. They may also boost inflammation; waist circumference greater than 40 inches in men and 35 inches in women. High waist circumference increases the risk for diabetes mellitus 2, dyslipidemia, HTN, and CVA in patients with BMI 25-34.9. BMI = height to weight ratio.

Stress management is a life skill. The danger of stress is that it can start to feel normal. Don't let it!

There is a phenomenon that can occur after nerve insult called spasticity. Spasticity involves muscle tension that doesn't release.

It can be devastating and painful when muscles over-respond. No matter the thoughts to relax, the position is held until an outside force intervenes via medicine or physical contact. That contact maneuvers the limb or joint into a state of relaxation.

Have you ever met an individual who is always on? It almost becomes a nuisance being in their presence. It can be painful or uncomfortable to see or feel the impact of constant talking, moving, and engaging. That person seems not to have the ability to shut off the constant action. Being aware of the tendency to always be on is the first step to finding a way to be at ease.

In any matter that needs fixing, the first step is to acknowledge the need to be fixed; whether being stressed with no hope of a way out or physically being addicted to a person or thing. One must acknowledge the problem and decide to get help. (The spastic muscle will NOT relax on its own while being stimulated). Help is available. Know that there is a solution even when the situation appears to be without hope. Hope deferred makes the heart sick. Change your mind and make the first step. Remember, you are wonderfully made for a purpose.

CHAPTER FOUR
Now What?

Knowing- it is said- is half the battle!

Just breathe, smell the roses! Stop for a moment and inhale through your nose, take in a full breath. Allow your abdomen to expand. Relax your shoulders and upper body.

Allow your diaphragm to contract. Sense the air coming in to bring needed oxygen. It will flow through your body to be used to energize and fuel you. Allow your mind to sense your cells' anticipation of wellbeing. Change your mind and don't mind your belly protruding out. This is for you, for your wellbeing.

Now, let it out. Purse your lips and allow the air to flow out. Blow out the candles, the waste, that which you don't need. Release the old, the unnecessary. Keep your shoulders relaxed. No stress, just deep breathing. Deeply be aware of the power to be in control of this air circulating in and out. In with the necessary and out with the unnecessary.

I have seen and experienced the evidence of deep breathing's effectiveness. Patients whose oxygen saturation levels (how much oxygen they were receiving) were low, changed from levels of concern to normal levels. The patient has been able to watch the monitor and see the oxygen level rise. When just starting to exercise and being winded and trying to "catch my breath," I have used this technique. Deep breathing is effective even at the gym! It's even more effective because I'm aware that I'm changing my levels by knowing the effectiveness before I even start. Here's how it works.

Lungs are our fuel tanks. Oxygen is the body's life-sustaining gas; it's breathed in then passed into our blood, then to tissues and organs. It is necessary for us to exist. It supplies cells with energy. When we breathe out, we produce carbon dioxide. The lungs take in about 2000 gallons of air each day. It provides oxygen to the blood that is pumped daily by the heart.

As air is breathed in through the nose, the nasal hairs act as a filter and trap dust. The air is warmed by the many blood vessels in the nasal membranes before passing through the windpipe. Air travels through the bronchi, then to the alveoli. It is there that important gas exchange takes place.

Oxygen passes from the alveoli to the capillaries to the heart then to the cells. Deoxygenated blood is returned to be oxygenated. Carbon dioxide - the waste product travels out of the blood to be eliminated. The brain controls the rate of our breathing and is sensitive to changes in gases. This is important because the brain is the biggest user of oxygen.

The diaphragm - muscles between the chest and abdomen is essential in our breathing pattern. The muscles contract when we breathe in, enlarging the lungs and letting in air. When we breathe out, the diaphragm relaxes, and the lungs deflate.

Deep breathing is an excellent relaxation tool. It can be practiced sitting or lying down. Simply slowly breathe in through your nose, relaxing your shoulders and allow your lower abdomen to protrude. Breathe in to a slow count of four. Purse your lips like you are about to blow out a candle and slowly blow out to a count of four.

The goal is to take in as much fresh air/oxygen from the lungs into the abdomen. The more oxygen, the less tense you feel. Practice with a hand or book on your belly and feel it rise as you bring air in, and fall as you breathe out. Music and aromatherapy can enhance the experience.

As mentioned earlier in the stress topic, when over-whelmed, our body is flooded with stress hormones which cause you to react with fight or flight. Everyday life stressors can wear the body down and take an exacting toll. There is a relaxation response that does the opposite of the stress response.

The relaxation response:

- Decreases the heart rate
- Allows breathing to become deeper and slower
- Blood pressure drops
- Muscles relax
- Blood flow to the brain increases

Practicing relaxation is essential. Knowing the feeling of tensed muscles allows you to relax them consciously.

Muscle relaxation involves tensing and relaxing muscle groups. As mentioned, with practice you become familiar with what tension and total relaxation feel like throughout the body. As you feel yourself starting to tense, you can choose to relax by letting go of that tension. This process will happen quicker and easier as it becomes a part of your norm.

It is important to practice one muscle group at a time. You can choose to start at your head and work down to your feet or vice versa. (Check with your physician to be sure muscle tension is not contraindicated for you).

> At the neck: tuck your chin down, resist the motion and feel the tension in the front of your neck, hold 3 secs, then fully let go.

> Tilt your head back, resist the motion, hold 3 secs. then release; tilt your head sideways, resist, hold , and release; repeat on the opposite side.

> At the shoulders, elevate your shoulders like you're indicating "I don't know." Hold 3 seconds, then relax.

> Bend your elbow fully, then with the opposite hand try to straighten it just enough to feel tension, then let go. Straighten the elbow, try to bend it with the opposite hand, then let go.

> Bend your knee up to your chest and hold it there while trying to push it down with your hand just enough to feel tension. Repeat on the opposite side.

> Straighten your knee fully and tighten your quadricep muscle, hold 3 seconds, then relax fully. Repeat on the opposite side.

> Bend your knee back fully, feel the tension, hold, then relax. Repeat on the opposite side.

> Bend your ankles up fully, feel the tension, then relax.

> Crunch forward as to tighten your abdominal muscles, hold, then relax.

> Ball your fingers into a tight fist then relax.

These exercises are to familiarize you with tension throughout your body. As you learn your body's feelings of tension, you can counter act that feeling with relaxation. They are not intended to cause any pain or discomfort. If any pain is felt, stop immediately and consult your doctor.

I have seen and personally experienced the power of deep breathing and the benefits of relaxation techniques. During gym workouts, deep breathing has allowed me to finish the task successfully. I surprise myself sometimes when I find my shoulders tense and I have to remind myself to relax. They are powerful tools to de-stress and empower our lives.

Conclusion

Relaxation should be purposeful. It is a choice to react in a manner that leaves you in control. Practicing being weightless (relaxed) becomes habitual and a natural state. Some people find confidence in a Type A persona, though one can still be on and yet relaxed.

Choose to silence the negative thoughts that come your way by resisting them. This can be done by actually speaking the words I rebuke it or I resist the thought. With regular resistance, they indeed will go away. Words are powerful. Do not accept ones that don't build you up. Step away from the noise.

If you are struggling to find your reason why, your purpose, look for your footprints. They will lead you. They will reinforce you. They'll give you a foundation to build on!

Out of the heart, the mouth speaks. Speak life!

Now that you're informed, what's next? Having the blueprint in hand, knowing the layout, and having the material for the project does not automatically cause the project to exist.

Someone must start the building. Once given the go-ahead (license to build), if the builder doesn't start, the building will not manifest. Contractors will be ready but awaiting the call to arrive at the building site. Someone must take the initiative to start. Materials management may be standing ready with the supplies. They need to be told we are ready for you to bring the items. You must now move forward. Just Do It. Do it with confidence. Each step, each decision involves you. You are the foreman, the boss, and the CEO. Others' lives will be enhanced by your decision to go. Be inspired. Be courageous. Make choices to be the better you than previously. You are wonderfully made. Know it and know it well!

For Your Inspiration

Numbers 6:26, "The Lord look over you and give you peace."

The very source of peace is the Lord. He watches us and releases peace. It is up to us to receive it.

Psalm 34:14, "Turn away from evil and do good; seek peace and pursue it."

Do good rather than evil. Search for the peaceful way out.

Psalm 122:6, "Pray for the peace of Jerusalem. May all who love this city prosper."

A prayer that peace will rule where God is honored, Prosperity for those who love and celebrates Jerusalem.

Colossians 3:15, "Let the peace of Christ rule in your hearts, since as members of one body you were called to peace. And be thankful."

Let peace be in your heart, it is a choice that is up to you. It calls out to you. Be thankful and let it.

Hebrews 12:14, "Make every effort to live in peace with everyone and to be holy."

Your focus to be at peace with those who you come into contact with results in you being at peace.

1 Peter 5:7, "Cast all your anxiety on Him because he cares for you."

You don't have to carry the load. You are loved and cared for. Find comfort in that and let go of anxious thoughts.

Philippians 4:7, "And the peace of God, which transcends all understanding, will guard your hearts and your minds in Christ Jesus."

Peace of God in your heart and mind can manifest in ways beyond what we can understand.

Proverbs 12:20, "Those who promote peace have joy."

Result of pushing the agenda of peace is that it brings joy with it.

1 Peter 3:10,11, "Whoever would love life and see good days must keep their tongue from evil and their lips from deceitful speech. Turn from evil and do good, seek peace and pursue it."

The natural impulse to return harshness with harshness will not bring peace. Turn away from deception even though it may be alluring. Choose good, follow hard after peace.

Philippians 4:6, "Do not be anxious about anything, but in every situation, by prayer and petition with thanksgiving present your requests to God."

Don't worry about anything. Pray with thanksgiving. Bring your concerns to the problem solver.

Psalm 119:165, "Great peace have those who love your law, and nothing can make him stumble."

If you love God, you will obey Him. He orders your steps, therein is great peace.

References

Stroke risks (2017) www.americanstrokeassociation.org

(2017) www.americanheartassosciation.org

Cohen Janson Barbara and Hull L. Kerry (2009) Structure and Function of the Human Body.

(2018) www.biblestudytools.com

For Contact/ Bookings:

Dorshena M. Pittman

www.theptforyou.com

theptforyou@gmail.com

PO Box 481 Destrehan, La. 70047

www.ingramcontent.com/pod-product-compliance
Lightning Source LLC
Chambersburg PA
CBHW071141280326
41935CB00010B/1316